What a monumental and genuine expression of endearing love, ultimate faithfulness, with the hope of triumphant Glory that a son has for his father! Truly, the Lord has divinely blessed the author of this book, as He will surely bless each reader who opens the cover of this magnificent, inspirational, true-to-life, literary work.

—Robert L. Heichberger, Ph,D.
Distinguished Professor Emeritus,
State University of New York

It is an outstanding narrative of life, and it is truly *"about a relationship between father and son communicating in silence with their souls in communion with their eternal Creator."* It demonstrates unconditional love and an attempt to understand ourselves. Thanks for the opportunity to read the book and digest the meaning!

—Ernie
Chair, Department of Management
Curry College, Milton, Massachusetts

The book is a powerful tool for others navigating this horrible disease. ...That Alzheimer's cannot "blemish" the soul was such a beautiful message to close with and help others to communicate and navigate their way through this disease with great calm and acceptance.

—Jacqui Namaste
EYRT (Experienced Registered Yoga Teacher), Master Yoga Life Coach, Director of Sacred Seeds Yoga School (RYS), Boston, Massachusetts.

As the executive director and chief executive officer of The Alzheimer's Association of Central Ohio, I have seen the devastating effects that Alzheimer 's disease has on those diagnosed with Alzheimer's and those that care for them. It's not just the people with Alzheimer's who suffer. It is also their caregivers. This book was written for you, the caregiver.

Alzheimer's robs people of their memories, their ability to communicate with loved ones and friends, and their ability to recognize their own image; it takes away our very soul. It is the cruelest of all diseases. John has experienced what you are going through; all the guilt, frustration, anger and hopelessness which makes this book an invaluable guide for you to follow. This book is about hope!

By reading this book you'll discover a method of communication that will help you maintain a meaningful relationship with your loved one.

—Kenneth E. Strong, Jr.
Upper Arlington, Ohio

NURTURING

LOVE

THROUGH THE SILENCE

NURTURING

LOVE

THROUGH THE SILENCE

LIVING WITH ALZHEIMER'S

JOHN DICICCO

TATE PUBLISHING
AND ENTERPRISES, LLC

Published by Tate Publishing & Enterprises, LLC
127 E. Trade Center Terrace | Mustang, Oklahoma 73064 USA
1.888.361.9473 | www.tatepublishing.com

Tate Publishing is committed to excellence in the publishing industry. The company reflects the philosophy established by the founders, based on Psalm 68:11,
"The Lord gave the word and great was the company of those who published it."

Book design copyright © 2011 by Tate Publishing, LLC. All rights reserved.
Cover design by Kate Stearman
Interior design by Christina Hicks

Published in the United States of America

ISBN: 978-1-61346-974-3
1. Health & Fitness / Diseases / Alzheimer's & Dementia
2. Religion / Christian Life / Inspirational
11.11.17

Dedication

I dedicate this book to my mother,
Filomena A. DiCicco
&
in memory of my father,
Ralph Joseph DiCicco senior

As it reads on his place of rest,
"Loving Husband, Father and Grandfather."
His legacy lives on.

Acknowledgments

I would like to thank Dr. Richard Leverault, physician, colleague, and friend, for showing me the way.

I want to remember a very dear friend, Anthony Pino, who recently passed away at the writing of this book. He was a gentleman, neighbor, and like a second father to me growing up. He too was lost to Alzheimer's and now joins my dad in eternal life.

Table of Contents

Introduction

My connection with Dad especially over the past five and one half years has been an astounding journey of learning about my humanity through Dad's inner being, his soul. This connection was a journey of unconditional love, guided with faith, and nurtured with deep appreciation for why we share this gift we call life. The interesting part of this journey was that it never began or ended with Dad's physical passing. It was my level of consciousness that was raised confirming the essence of his spiritual self. The journey continued with his soul as his physical life was coming to an end. Yes, Dad's humanity and the physical end to it confirmed my earlier convictions that the soul is eternal and lives on despite physical death. The soul has no beginning and no end. It just is.

I am convinced that the soul lives on, and memory alone is not what keeps Dad alive forever. You see, the essence of being has no past or future. Only what is exists. Spiritual consciousness of the connection between one human being and another bonded through unconditional love seeks no retribution, no consequences, and certainly no justification. It just is.

Alzheimer's disease robs the human brain of its ability to remain in the conscious world a little bit more each day, each month, and each year until the person dies. I know this to be true as I watched Dad's brain lose its ability to guide and control what his body needed to sustain his day-to-day functioning. However, what I did clearly see was my increased ability to communicate with his true inner being, his soul. Dad's soul is what made Dad *Dad*. His soul communicated with my soul in ways that I could never have imagined. I learned about him in the silence of raised consciousness most intensely in the last six months of his physical life when his soul embraced consciousness as one with God. I will refer to God going forward in this book as "the eternal Creator."

I felt compelled to write this book about Dad and his journey living with a human disease called "Alzheimer's." I wish to give hope to all who suffer with this affliction or who live with one afflicted with this horrible and dreaded infirmity. This book is written to convince those who fear Alzheimer's to take a journey with it and learn that unconditional love accepts and embraces human frailty and glorifies the soul. We grow spiritually through the silence, and the silence eases our pain while diminishing our fears.

As I write this book, I am guided by the hand of the eternal Creator of all things who, through his love and wisdom, inspired me to share in the magnificent wonder of the human soul. This is the soul that replicates the Creator in his image and likeness and delivers a clear message of hope and a true sense of comfort during this physically and emotionally painful journey.

Finally, this book is not about my life or Dad's life. Rather, it is about a relationship between father and son communicating in silence with their souls with their eternal Creator who makes all things possible through of unconditional love. This period in which I write is where spirituality becomes a reality, an absolute of our combined existence defining a special communion with our Creator. This communion does not seek any validation, conviction, or justification. It requires no words. It does require much silence and reflection.

Letting Go of the Human Connection

When we lose a loved one, we suffer great emotional pain, and this is why it is paramount to understand and accept divine existence during human loss. When we accept the soul as eternal and always existing in the present, emotion can also provide a gateway to the soul. Pain is only temporary in this life when we believe that the soul is eternal and without physical or emotional pain. The majority of what is to come in this book when defining or addressing the soul will be written in the present tense as the soul always is and is not in any time continuum we define as past or future. I started my thinking this way initially as a source of comfort from some very dreaded emotions that were wretched and dark, to put it mildly. Alienating oneself from physical pain is self-preserving and natural.

In mid-morning on May 2, 2010, as I watched Dad's human life come to an end with my family during every struggling breath he took, I was continuing my spiritual journey with him and not ending it. I may have not realized this consciously at the time, but I felt it in my soul. I later understood what I felt at that time when I became more aware of a richer, much more rewarding experience than I could ever imagine while focusing on spiritual connectivity rather than physical loss.

Most readers of this book may believe that thinking in terms of getting through the pain of losing the physical connection with the human body of the loved one represents an inner strength and is normally accepted as part of the grieving process. Honestly, I really thought this too until three weeks before Dad's passing when I went for my annual physical with my primary care physician. I have known this doctor for about twenty years and trust him implicitly. I told him about the grave situation Dad was in physically and that he had only a few weeks left before his human life would come to an end. I told the doctor I was devastated by this news and refused to accept that there were no other options available to save his life. This doctor had always comforted me and given me strength. This doctor was the most compassionate individual I have ever known.

The doctor looked at me intensely and said, "John, is this about you or about your father?" I did not know how to respond to his question. I was speechless. Here I was speaking to the most compassionate guy in the world, and he turned this around one hundred eighty degrees. I never looked at the situation this way, and it threw me completely. His comment was completely out of character for him, as it appeared as if the voice of the Creator was speaking through him. I then realized that I was dealing with my physical loss of Dad's human connectivity to me and how I would feel about living with that loss. Also, this was not about me and not even about Dad. This was about our relationship once his body ceased to function.

After leaving the doctor's office, I then realized how selfish I had been. I was focused so much on losing Dad that I completely forgot to remember our spiritual connection over the past five and a half years. I forgot what I had learned about him as a person whose thoughts and emotions I shared. I was more focused on my painful emotions while watching him die that I didn't consider how he would feel if he knew I was suffering so much in the process.

In retrospect, if this were the case then the time that I had spent with him over the past five and a half years was in vain. The only thing that I could think about at this time was how I spent day after day wondering what type of physical or mental states he would be in. Would he be choking on his own saliva? Would he not be able to breathe on his own? Would he not be able to pass his urine, or would he come down with another episode of the C-DiF?

I knew that the end would be here soon. I had to prepare myself mentally and physically for what was to come; would I be able to handle it? Again, I was thinking more of how this would affect me more than how it would affect Dad as he watched me feel his weakened essence. My fears began to rise once again, and my emotions heightened. I became bitter, confused, and angered by thoughts that focused on losing him. Yes,

I was being selfish, once again. I did not know what to do or how to feel. I became bitter and alienated to the point where I found it difficult to function without thinking about losing Dad. I did not know whether to talk to a priest or seek psychological assistance. I needed guidance, and I needed it now.

I remember shortly after my return to work, on my desk there was a book. One of my colleagues placed it on my desk. The book was entitled *Conversations with God, an Uncommon Dialogue, Book 1*. I briefly skimmed through the pages and did not immediately make the connection as to why it was left for me to read. I returned to my daily activities and then picked up the book once again. And as I flipped through the pages, I realized that there was a purpose behind my receiving this book at this time. I just did not know why.

At the day's end, I approached my colleague and asked why she gave me this book to read. She explained to me that several years ago one of her dear friends told her to read the book and how inspirational it was for her to understand certain things about her purpose in being born to this earth and, most importantly, her relationship with her Creator. My colleague then explained to me that she thought of me as she was doing some general cleaning in her house and discovered the book, which she had not seen for quite some time. She thought it might help me get through this difficult period. I thanked her and put the book aside, figuring that I would read it later on.

The next three weeks became increasingly difficult for me to cope with. As I watched Dad's condition continue to deteriorate, I became increasingly angered and confused. My physical and mental state was also rapidly deteriorating to the point that I dreaded the next day. I prayed feverishly for guidance. I was filled with grief and despair and asked for a miracle to keep Dad alive. Suddenly my doctor's voice resounded through my being. I remembered him saying to me, "Are we being a little selfish here, John? Is this about you or about your dad?"

When I arrived home, I began to read the book that my colleague had given me. At first I was apprehensive but found the dialogue in the book intriguing. I began to feel some comfort in what I was reading as my awareness and understanding of what was happening around me began to make sense. It did not make sense from a religious standpoint but rather from a spiritual one. As I continued to read, it became increasingly obvious that there was a distinct difference between faith and religion. I now found comfort in helping Dad in his journey, which would lead to the end of his physical life as we know it.

In the last five-plus years, I have begun to remember Dad in a very special way, in a very spiritual way, experiencing the ultimate connection that we refer to as "unconditional love."

Unconditional love does not require a prerequisite or a resume. It has no beginning and no end. Yet it is the alpha and omega of all existence. Although we may never be able to understand it, we know it exists. The eternal silence of the soul speaks with incredible passion and is such a complete love that it holds no boundaries that are exhibited through human frailty. Concrete evidence of unconditional love cannot be validated yet cannot be ignored. We all know it exists because we feel it but cannot explain it. This is our connection to the soul that is, that was, and will always be an infinite manifestation larger than the universe and smaller than the smallest pinhead at the same time. Understanding this concept is part of our divine dichotomy that we will understand when we enter eternal life through our souls without human frailty. My emotions were now ready to accept that Dad's physical life was coming to an end. His physical life ended, and his spiritual life continued at approximately seven forty p.m., May 3, 2010.

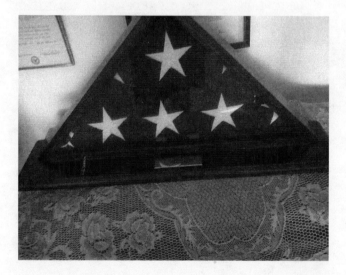

Knowing Dad through the Human Connection

On May 7, 2010, I opened Dad's eulogy by relating his responses to my mother when she woke him up in the middle of the night to tell him that she had to go to the hospital. This occurred on the evening of November 4, 1951. Dad's response to mother was, "What is the matter? Are you sick?"

Mother's response to Dad was "I am having a baby!"

I guess you could say that this was the beginning of my relationship with my father. Dad was a loving and gentle man and always looked at life with a lot of humor. Yet he took his life very seriously when it came to taking care of his wife and children. In every way he would offer hope to every decision that he made. I know that this is a very awkward thing to say. Usually one would expect love, and not hope, to be the underlying motivation behind making decisions in most instances.

The best way to describe a human relationship would be to accept the divine dichotomy as truth to the relationship that exists between the body and the soul during the course of earthly life. Love, described as a human emotion, is much different than unconditional love, which emanates the soul. However, the divine dichotomy, which connects the soul and the body through our five earthly senses, allows us in our humanity to experience the human emotion of love in mortal terms. I never consciously realized this until I began my journey with Dad, beginning almost seven years ago when he was diagnosed with a terrible affliction referred to as "Alzheimer's disease." In the last five and a half years of Dad's earthly existence, I spent almost every day watching his human body slowly deteriorate as a result of this disease. I asked the divine Creator why he was putting me through this terrible suffering and why was he punishing me by allowing me to watch Dad slowly die. I began to resent my relationship with my father because I hated to go to the veterans' administration hospital where he was being treated and watch him die a little more each day.

I often wondered why God was punishing me by allowing me to see my father lose a little bit more of what I remembered him to be. I began to blame God for putting me through this terrible affliction. The affliction I am referring to was my own emotional pain and not Dad's inability to communicate with me within a relationship that was natural for me. I simply did not understand. Bitterness and resentment consumed me each day I visited Dad. I needed to change my attitude but did not have a justification to do so during this very difficult time in my life, living with Alzheimer's disease.

I found this part of the human connection to be very challenging. I had a very different opinion of how mental anguish should be handled. I remembered that when I was a child, Dad would take me on his shoulders and walk me through the Boston Common as we headed to the Swan boats without having a care in the world. I cannot specifically remember who was there, how old I was, what was around me, or how the water from the manmade lake splashed on my face while Dad and I were laughing and enjoying ourselves on the Swan boats. The point is, every time I think of that time together, I can still feel the love and emotion that consumed me many decades ago. I believe I can still feel that love because it came from the soul, which consumed my body, and that love is not bound by time.

Connecting my experiences with Dad on the swan boats many years ago and feeling the same way now just as I remember them defines the limitless boundaries of unconditional love.

I often observe faith and religion in the same vein. I find that religion is very consequential. And there are certain steps that must be taken and obeyed to achieve the ultimate bliss or joy that I refer to as "unconditional love."

Growing up as a Roman Catholic, I often remember how I was taught to believe in God, Jesus, and the Holy Spirit. I was taught to believe that there were three persons in one God. This was the mystery of our faith. The point is that we were taught not to question or understand this sacred mystery. In my entire life, I could never understand how it was possible for three entities to co-exist simultaneously and all as part of each other, having very different roles for one another. In holy mass, we recite the "mystery of our faith." We all pray together, "Christ has died. Christ has risen. Christ will come again." It appears apparent to me this "mystery of faith" is something that cannot be explained. My question is, how can you die a mortal death and then rise from the dead after human life ceases to continue? We cannot understand this in human terms. Our faith is what saves us and brings us to a higher conscious level, where we can appreciate the mysteries of faith, where they lie and not where they originate. I also believe that what exists in God and in God's eyes exists in us and in all our eyes if we are willing to see through the windows of unconditional love. God is unconditional love, and we are made in his image and likeness.

As I watched Dad deteriorating in his human body, I was unaware that at a higher-conscious level he was reaching me without saying a word. He appeared to be talking to me with his eyes. Often telepathic communications cannot be explained in words but are felt through our emotions. In my case, it was simply felt as a communication of unconditional love between father and son. His eyes were not necessarily sad but rather expressive to me in a very personal way. At the Brockton VA hospital when I was looking at Dad's eyes, none of the nurses or nurses' assistants saw or felt what I did when I looked into Dad's eyes. Although

John DiCicco

these nurses cared passionately for Dad's well being, they could not rationalize nor understand what I saw and felt when I looked into his eyes. This felt emotion was and still is part of me as it is part of him in life and death. As we know, it is simply "the human connection" guided through the spiritual soul.

Knowing is not the same as learning. As an educator, I know that learning is based on observation and facts. On the other hand, knowing may not always be based on facts and is often based on intuition.

I am very analytical and have been trained to think scientifically and not emotionally. However, I have been stopped in my tracks at this point of my life and have felt an urgent, compelling need to write this book. I say this with great humility and feel comfort through this book in helping me understand the true nature of unconditional love. My experience dealing with my dad's Alzheimer's has opened my life to a whole different meaning and a higher conscious level of why I exist and that I really never lost Dad from a spiritual viewpoint. Finally, I realized that Dad was and is part of me and will always be part of me, as I am part of the Creator, as the Creator is part of both Dad and me. I did not choose to rationalize this or understand this from my limited human knowledge. However, I feel it, and what I feel I want to share to give those who are experiencing terrible emotional pain, watching their loved ones or learning for the first time about them having been diagnosed with Alzheimer's, that the human connection of their existence at one point will be lost and will never return to them. However, the spiritual connection will live on for eternity.

Seeing Beyond the Human Connection

As a child, while still in elementary school, I would often wonder what purpose I had to be born to this earth. At this very young age, I questioned my own existence. My thoughts made me feel quite strange, and they frightened me. I never shared this with anyone because I thought they would think there was something wrong with me. I thought my friends would laugh at me or ridicule me for these thoughts. I never shared them with my parents because this is not what elementary school students thought of, especially when I was a child. As I grew through my teenage years, these thoughts never left me. In fact, they continued to grow stronger.

I attended a Catholic elementary school in my pre-teen years and a Catholic high school in my teenage years. My religious values were strongly reinforced at home and in my education. My upbringing taught me never to question my religious values. My strict

Catholic upbringing made me fear these values more than love what they represented as I continued to learn and grow and mature in the world around me. My mother taught me that love of family and of each other within that family held a very special place in God's eyes. My mother taught me to love God more than fear him. However, my religion always taught me that the fear of God would get me into heaven and the love of God would save me from going to hell. These values caused great conflict in my mind and often made me question my purpose in being born to this world. What was I supposed to accomplish? What difference does it make whether or not I exist? Again, these were very frightening thoughts. I thought I was losing my mind and often blocked these thoughts out when they became too severe.

I remembered that my strict religious upbringing reinforced the fact that I had a soul and my body was a temple of the Holy Spirit. I was also taught that my soul was born with a blemish, which is called "original sin." I never could understand why I was born with sin on my soul. And I had this blemish on my soul before I was even born into human existence. However I never questioned my religion as my parents taught me. I was told that Adam and Eve committed a grave sin many years before I was born. I often wondered why I was being punished for something that they did. I was told by my religious educators that everyone born into this world had this blemish on their souls and must repent. Our human existence would be judged on how we live our lives. Original sin would never go away.

It is eminently clear to me at this point that religion, whatever that religion is, builds an awareness of spiritualism that provides construct and purpose to the soul. I am okay with that and continue to respect the traditions and values of my religious upbringing and what it has taught me. It does, however, open to us all an opportunity to raise our thinking and spiritual awareness to a higher level of consciousness.

I want to clarify that *consciousness* and *awareness* in spiritual terms may not be the same thing. One can be very conscious but not very aware of the impact that the body and the soul of one human being are connecting with the body and the soul of another human being. In the five years plus that I visited Dad almost every day at the Brockton veterans' hospital, my connection with him in physical terms was getting less and less as far as cognition was concerned, considering his physical level of awareness in his surrounding environment. However, his response time to my enthusiastic greetings made me more aware of his spiritual consciousness, and more sensitive to the lack of his physical consciousness. Having said this, I needed to redefine my purpose in visiting him each day. Some days after visiting Dad, I would shake my head, look up to the sky, and ask God why he was making me do this day after day. I would feel incredibly guilty if I did not visit Dad each day. I felt he looked forward to seeing me, although his physical response and awareness to my visits continued to diminish, especially in the last two years of his physical life.

I needed to clarify my spiritual connection with my Dad and not ponder on the fact that he would die soon. Unless this mandate was met, I could not continue to emotionally handle continued visits with Dad. The spiritual aspects to which I refer are broken down into several components as described by name in the chapters to follow. Each component of spirituality will represent a special correlation of the connectedness of the human soul of one human being at a higher level of consciousness to the human soul of another human being. "Physical degradation" refers to the continued deteriorating state of my father's human body as Alzheimer's disease progressed with each successive time I visited the Brockton veterans' hospital.

Throughout my life, I often wondered how God could allow people to suffer with terrible pain. I also wondered how God could allow people to die in earthquakes or turn his back on a little baby drowning in the bathtub while his mother walks away to answer a telephone call or on an entire family getting buried under a mud slide after a severe rainstorm. I had no answers to any of this and figured I would find out after my human life ended. I often asked my dad these questions as I was growing up. He said he really did not have an answer and said that there must be a good reason. Then he simply changed the subject. This was Dad—short, sweet, and to the point. Dad never really pondered on any one thing for too long. However, he lived a simple, meaningful existence throughout his human life.

In retrospect, Dad's wisdom portrayed an incredible message to me. He may not have consciously been aware of this, but he simply knew what to say. In the last two years of Dad's life, the silence of which I refer to in the title of this book made a very loud spiritual noise. The noise may have been louder than any earthquake or explosion. The silence of the human condition at a lower level of consciousness is heard by all and often simply ignored. Dad's silence as his disease progressed and made room for the beautiful sounds that were to be heard at a higher level of consciousness.

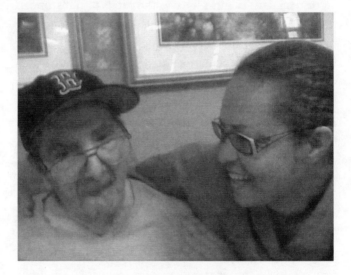

At a higher level of consciousness, the sound is not heard through the vibration of molecules that enter the ear canal as experienced by the human mind. Rather, the sound is the manifestation of all knowledge that answers many of my questions. The interesting point here is that I did not realize any of this until May 3, 2010, at Dad's funeral mass. Suddenly all became clear to me that his whole life was a message of unconditional love. To those who know him, he was just a simple, ordinary human being and who did the best he could to live a good life.

Just before his casket left the church, held high by the pallbearers on its way to his final resting place, I was incredibly sad. Almost instantly this feeling of incredible sadness was replaced with exuberant, indescribable joy. I could not even understand my own emotions, let alone deal with them. This was the catalyst that stopped me in my tracks and made me decide to not waste any time and write this book. I felt I needed to share this wonderful experience and put it into words and provide comfort and understanding to all those who may have a loved one that is experiencing the dreaded affliction of Alzheimer's disease or have just been recently diagnosed with the disease. This book is not about closure of a dreaded human experience. Rather, it is about the acknowledgment of incredible communication with the human soul that holds no boundaries, offers no forgiveness, requires no retribution for sins committed, and speaks only of eternal life. I now realize that my earthly existence recognizes eternal life and is one with it rather than separate from it throughout earthly humanity.

Rationalizing eternal life as coexisting with human life is extremely difficult. It is even more difficult to raise human consciousness that experiences both mind and spirit as one rather than separate. Yoga or meditation may help the human body recognize you as one with your eternal soul. In the absence of any deep meditative thought during the last two years of Dad's life, I was able to see beyond the human connection, without meditation or yoga, and communicate with his soul. I got to know him for who he really was and realized he was me and I was him. I also realized that Dad and I communicated with the eternal Creator. In my mind, this represented unconditional love that requires no validation for its existence and provides for the deep meaning of why we exist, rather than how we exist as one entity. I also realized that unconditional love has no past or future. Only the present is what counts. This is different than living for the moment and only existing for the present experience. Rather, it is a connection that delineates the human soul as eternal with the eternal Creator.

In my strict Roman Catholic upbringing, I was always taught that God and I were separate and we needed to pay for sins and repent in order to get to heaven and be one with God. In January of 2008 when Dad's physical condition began to deteriorate at an increasingly rapid pace, I truly began my journey with his soul in communion with my soul.

Understanding the Human Connection

"With him and in him in the unity of the Holy Spirit all glory and honor is yours, oh, almighty Father, forever and ever." This is a part of the holy Catholic mass that I repeated with Dad Sunday after Sunday while attending mass with him in the last two years of his human life. These words in this part of the mass follow the consecration of the Eucharist in the most holy part of the mass. I was educated and nurtured to believe that ordinary bread and wine was changed into the body and blood of our Lord and Savior, Jesus Christ. These words clearly delineate a purpose of faith—humanity, and only humanity, represents the gateway to the soul. After the consecration in the holy Catholic mass, the priest will validate the human sacrifice of Christ's death by stating, "Do this in remembrance of me."

It is ever present in my mind that there is a distinct difference between faith and religion. Religion requires obedience, and faith requires love, resulting in obedience of choice. As a young Roman Catholic, I remember being taught that God gave us all free will to choose whether we would live a life of righteousness or a life of evil. If we chose the latter, the consequences would result in eternal damnation. However, we had the opportunity to repent for our sins a number of different ways, and God would absolve us through his everlasting forgiveness and love for us.

Getting back to Dad, I would like to talk about the relationship between Mom and Dad and the love they felt for each other. Notice that I used the word *felt*. To feel is to experience. To experience requires no validation. It just exists for the present. Feeling has no past and no future. Alzheimer's patients in their advanced stages seem to live only in the present, and what they remember, despite how long ago, is always in the present. Watching Dad for the last two years of his human life, having only the ability to remember what occurred in the past gave me a better understanding of how through faith such a physically devastating disease could provide a strong spiritual comfort from the unconditional love that exists between an inflicted loved one and a connected family member.

"Do this in memory of me." This quotation represents much more than words, as it relates to Christ's message when he sat with his disciples at the last supper. "Memory" now takes on a whole meaning for purposes of this narrative. I speak of faith and not religion. Whether one believes or not that bread and wine are changed into the body and blood of Jesus Christ, I want to focus on the word *memory*. Attending mass every Sunday with Dad and watching him observe the priest and not be able to fully recite all the words of the Our Father prayer was a real challenge for me emotionally. As a kid growing up, attending mass with him on Sunday, he championed the Our Father with ease by reciting every word without any prompting.

As his disease progressed in the last few years of his life while attending mass at the veteran's hospital, he failed to recite more and more words to the Our Father. His lips would quiver as he was trying to form the words but his muscles would not cooperate. He would stare at me and he appeared to be afraid. He would say nothing. He then gave up and stopped trying because it drained every bit of energy from him just to continue with the prayer. He would then close his eyes tightly and settle in his wheelchair until he became unresponsive to any external stimulation. He appeared to be sleeping but was not. Then he would open his eyes and look at me with such helplessness. His left hand would be clenched tightly against his chest while his right lay limp against the railing of the wheelchair. Dad looked at me with confusion as if to ask, "What comes next?"

I would look at him with tenderness while on the inside I was plagued with mixed emotions of fear, anger, and humiliation of others observing his behavior at mass while he sat there, totally helpless. Many times he would be unresponsive to support by the nursing staff. Then, often times after mass ended, suddenly without any prompting he would look at me and begin to laugh. His wide smile radiated through my being and lifted my emotions to an all-time high. You see, we connected in silence not in words.

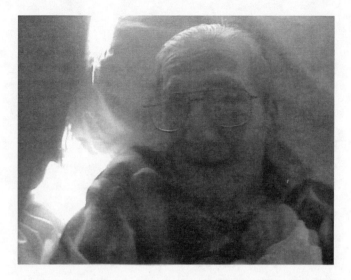

This connection brought me back to a time when we shared precious moments that didn't involve dialogue or a special place. This connection was a bonding that represented unconditional love between father and son. Therefore the painful memory of Dad forgetting the words to the Our Father was replaced by the wonderful memory of Dad's laughter in times when he was lucid. The key point is that he was smiling at me now just as he smiled many years ago, long before he was inflicted with this dreaded disease. The point is that my observation and his experience were at different levels of consciousness. The mass itself lasted no more than twenty minutes each Sunday morning. However, I did experience a very special connection to him.

Differentiating between the human and the divine connection was no longer challenging; it was next to impossible. The rationale behind this was that the connection was felt as one mind, body, and spirit. The human connection in finite terms deals with love as a word used to define so many different feelings or experiences. Many of these feelings are experiences that cannot be defined in words but are expressed verbally to show some form of affection. In the last five years of Dad's life, when visiting him at the Brockton Veterans' Hospital, I cannot remember a time when I did forget to say to him, "I love you." When I told him I loved him, it was irrelevant whether there were many people around us or we were alone. However, how those who may have heard these three words may have been very different from how Dad heard them. In fact, to take it one step farther, although his wide smile or his blank stare looking away from my face as I uttered these three words, "I love you," each day emotionally made me feel he was still hanging in there because of that unconditional love connection.

It is virtually impossible, especially in the last two years of his human life, to know whether or not he understood the three words "I love you." From my perspective, what appeared to be true was that Dad felt these words throughout his being, which cannot be explained by rational human thought as we know it to be. I call this "nurturing love through silence."

I remember one Sunday when my brother was in town with his wife to visit Dad, and he took my mother with them on the visit. I was running some errands and told my brother I would go to the veteran's hospital and join them after I finished running the errands. When I arrived, Dad was in his room, all dressed and spiffy, sitting up in his wheelchair with his eyes clenched tightly shut, making circular movements with his hands. However, he was not responding at all to the family's requests for him to open his eyes and acknowledge they were there. My brother explained to me that they had been at the hospital for several hours and he was in the same position and doing the same thing as I observed when I walked in to his room, basically in his own world and non-responsive.

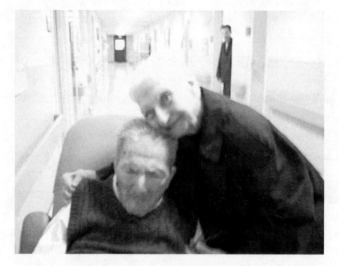

My family, including the staff, could not get Dad to respond to them with any type of acknowledgement they were there, even when they fed him. I looked at Dad with tenderness, and although his eyes were clenched shut, I felt something very emotional that I can't explain consume my being. This feeling startled me, and it felt like an electric shock going through my system. It was like pure positive energy that offered hope in the face of despair that I could connect with him.

I smiled at my family and went over to Dad's wheelchair and gently grabbed his hand that stopped making circular motions and softly whispered, "Dad, it's Johnny. How are you?"

His eyes were still tightly shut, and then suddenly he blurted out, "What?"

Gently, I stated once again, "It's Johnny. I am here. I love you!" I began stroking his arm and gently stroked his face. I stated again, this time a little louder in a more exuberant tone, "It's Johnny. I love you!" Suddenly he opened his eyes and looked at me and then began to laugh just as he did when we were at mass. Again, his wide smile lit up the room. My mom explained to my family that I saw him every day and he knew my voice. This may be true, but the connection I felt was unexplainable emotionally, and I believe it was much more than that he knew my voice. I believe it was the bond we shared at a higher spiritual level through unconditional love.

On several occasions on my daily visits to the Brockton Veterans' Hospital, my heart would be rapidly beating, my pulse would be elevated, and my mind would be filled with thoughts laced with fear. I would try to prepare myself for the worst news, that I would be told that Dad was very ill. As I walked through the double doors leading to Dad's room while bracing myself for the worst news, I often could breathe a sigh of relief when I saw Dad sitting up in his wheelchair, looking at me and smiling because he saw me. I then immediately rejected my fears for the time being and enjoyed my visit with Dad.

During my visit, I was not consciously aware of how long I was spending with Dad. Often my visit would not last more than five or ten minutes because I had to get ready for work right after my visit with him. However, all I needed was to see his smiling face and know that he was okay. This encounter was enough to bring me through the day and keep Dad's visual image of his smile in my mind throughout the day. In essence, I now realize that it was not the length of time that I spent with him that made a difference during my visit. Rather, it was what went on and what we both experienced during that time. In human terms, we refer to this as "quality time spent." In retrospect, during my visits, time and space had no bearing or influence in my communication with Dad. Rather than refer to this encounter with Dad as "quality time," this experience was timeless.

When I visited Dad, it was as if time stood still. Often when entering Dad's room, he appeared to be very confused as nurses assistants were cleaning him up and preparing him for breakfast. He was still in bed and not ready to get into his wheelchair. Often, the dementia would not allow him to open his eyes and see me. During these particular types of visits, Dad would be making circular motions with his hands and would be trying to move the muscles in his face so that he could say hello to me when I entered the room where he was being serviced. This type of behavior became more prevalent as the dementia continued to worsen.

The "human connection" between Dad and me became increasingly strained.

I felt like I was losing a little bit of him more each day, and what I observed was cruel and harsh, as it compromised his dignity and reduced his very being to a distorted replication of the man I once know. This man who could dance with the grace of Gene Kelly and who once possessed the wit of a polished comedian was deteriorating right before my eyes, and there was nothing I could do to stop it from happening! I watched his anguish as he tried to form words and then gave up after several attempts. I watched the wretched muscles quivering in his cheekbones and forehead as he attempted to say he loved me when I said good-bye and he tried to say it back. This special relationship that we built over a half century ago was quickly becoming a memory, and time was running out.

I remember one morning when I went to visit Dad and the nursing staff was trying to get him out of bed after cleaning him up. He was non-responsive with his eyes shut tight, and they told me they decided to keep him in bed, as he appeared tired and drained. I stayed by his bedside and tried to make conversation with him but to no avail. I then decided to leave and kissed him gently on the forehead, whispering, "It's Johnny. I love you!" He did not respond, so I left.

As I walked down the corridor toward the exit door of the veterans' hospital, I heard Dad say, "I love you too!" This was several minutes after I said that to him in his room. This is the connection of love that I can't explain or comprehend. I just know it happens and it exists because I felt it, heard it, and saw what it can do.

Thoughts of Dad carrying me through the Boston Common on his shoulders, laughing and smiling as we headed toward the Swan boats ran through my head. Watching him in this state, especially in the last year of his life, was extremely painful to say the least. When I was at a very young age, I had no inkling that I would be observing Dad in a hospital room at a nursing home where he could barely physically communicate with me. Even though half a century separated the extreme joy of the Swan boats from the extreme sadness of nursing home, I knew this passage of time was destiny. In other words, the two incidents mentioned above were transparent to one another, given that Dad in the normal course of time passage would be expected to end his natural life in a "normal" way. However, the human mind in a physical connection of extreme suffering on the part of the observer can only correlate extreme joy with extreme sorrow to justify the present experience, which is almost unbearable to view emotionally.

In retrospect what I learned was that my joyful experiences with Dad during the good times I shared with him in my youth did not mask the pain of watching him physically degenerate before my eyes. Rather, the memory of those good times provided comfort and hope on my part that Dad was thinking the same thing at a higher or different level of his spiritual existence until he took his last breath. In other words, his soul was communicating with mine through the instrument of unconditional love provided from our Eternal

Creator that would last beyond his last breath through eternity. This was not fully realized until I read my Dad's eulogy, which I wrote and shared at his funeral mass. I created an environment of self-serving pacification to my denial that I was slowly losing my father in a physical sense each time I visited him at the hospital. In essence, I was living in the world that did not prepare me for the end of Dad's natural life. Rather, I was living in environments that could only produce hope in my mind that Dad would continue his earthly existence in the state that I once knew him that referenced back to the time when he was carrying me on his shoulders to the Swan boats at a very young age. I was even willing to accept this continued deteriorating body as a substitute for these wonderful times. My selfishness was extreme, and I now realize in writing this book my visits to him were about me getting through this experience and not him.

Thoughts are influenced by values taught and values learned. My father taught me how to love, and he ingrained this value in my very being. The question that lies before me is, was I validating the love I had for my father when visiting him in his physically deteriorating state? Or was I trying to get a physical validation from Dad that he still could love me for my visiting him each day? Before Dad's dementia became so severe that he could not verbalize that he loved me, I could leave the hospital knowing that he felt toward me the way I felt toward him. Further, when the human connection in the physical sense was broken off or fragmented, I could not get that validation. I often would leave the nursing home, shaking my head and asking God why he was putting me through this experience. Again, this was all about me. I am not beating myself up here. I am not asking for forgiveness of what I felt or believed at the time of my visits. I needed some assurance that I was getting through to Dad. I needed to feel that spark of energy flowing through my body again that helped me make Dad open his tightly clenched eyes, look at me, and begin to laugh with a wide smile that lit up the room. It wasn't happening as the end drew near.

Suddenly, I remembered just a couple of weeks before Dad passed when he was almost totally unresponsive. A thought bubble emerged, and it all made sense. Well, it made sense to me at the time. I could not believe I forgot who I was. I was Dad's son. I did not need any other validation that he loved me. I did not need acceptance that he loved me by hearing him say it back or, even acknowledge it by his facial expressions. He didn't even have to move a muscle. Yes, he loved me unconditionally. I then remember looking at my hands and arms for some reason and realized this was all part of Dad. I am him and he is me. I am continuing his legacy by just being there for him. I was there for over five years, watching and learning from him how to love without judgment and how to cope with anguish through example by offering hope to others who are going through this same experience. Finally, I no longer needed to feel guilty of alienation from him when he was unresponsive. I was free from guilt and have always and will always be connected to him.

In the last two months of Dad's life, I could not bear the thought of losing him. I wrestled with the great conflict that existed in my mind between losing him forever and visiting him at the nursing home. I was becoming very irritable at work and unbearable to be with at home. I was not very pleasant to be around during this time. My work life and home life was not the same. I lived each dreaded day as if that day would be Dad's last. I snapped at co-workers if they spoke to me or shut them out completely if I had the chance. Some understood and some didn't at work. At home, I got a lot of compassion but that even goes away when you become unbearable to be with most times. I needed some type of closure but did not know how to validate that. At this time, I became angry at myself, angry at my family, angry at my work, and, most sadly, angry at my God for putting me through this horrific experience. This was so not me, and I desperately needed to change. I did not know how can I prayed to my creative for guidance.

I was becoming something that Dad would be ashamed of if he knew I was acting this way over him. Yes, it was all about me, and I couldn't stop it. I needed to pray for guidance before I lost my mind and my family. I did not know where to begin to pray. I always prayed for Dad to get well. I could not bear to pray for coping skills when he passed. I could not even bear the thought. I kept putting it off. However, I knew by the looks of things that the end would be coming soon. I needed to pray. Nothing else would offer me comfort or make me feel better.

At this point of my life, I was so focused, so obsessed with Dad's condition that I was oblivious to all of the support around me. I had to get a grip. I prayed for a sign that God didn't abandon me and assurance that Dad was not suffering. Deep down I didn't really understand what I was observing and tried to convince myself that I could make it okay. I always was able to fix things when they went wrong in the family. I couldn't fix what was happening to Dad, and I wanted to know why from God. I was angry, and I wanted so hard to lash out at Him and tell God He was making a mistake on Dad and should not take him now. You see, I still needed Dad, and I did not want to lose him because I knew that a part of me would die with him if he died. I frantically wanted to hold on to Dad's life because it would benefit me not Dad, and I didn't see it that way. I was too busy going to the nursing home or finding an excuse to know I still controlled whether he lived or died because only I could fix it. I didn't see that it was God's will not my will that decided when Dad could enter eternal life.

I asked God for a sign, and I got one. I went to my doctor for my annual physical, and he asked me if my concern with Dad was about me and not about Dad. At first, I was very offended that my doctor would ask me such a question. Having known him for almost twenty years, he was one of the gentlest, most compassionate people in my life. It was though something or someone else was talking through him and trying to send me a message. I have never been nor was I ever a supporter of mystical messages or superstitions. However,

I always felt that my faith was strong and that the Creator works in mysterious ways. My physical was on April 19, 2010. Dad passed away on May 3, 2010. I then realized that in order to get through losing Dad in his physical state, I needed to reach out and bring my level of consciousness to what I had been experiencing in my connection with him all along. This experience was not about my connection with his body, but rather my connection with his soul. This was my sign!

My realization at this point was that the only thing that would get me through losing Dad physically was to reconnect with him spiritually, which I had been doing all along in the five and a half years I had been visiting him at the nursing home. This experience would no longer be about me. Rather, it would be about Dad and me, and I would continue with our spiritual connection after his human connection ended. I was now ready for human closure, which I knew would be physically and emotionally painful to experience, yet was necessary. My religion teaches me. And my faith coincides with my mind, body, and spirit that Jesus, in order to reunite with his Father, the eternal Creator, needed to experience human death most tragically and painfully before he could holistically once again, in his true self, reunite with his Father.

Understanding the Spiritual Connection

I do not consider this to be a religious experience. However, I do believe this to be a spiritual journey, whereas my body is being used as an instrument of my eternal soul to express my thoughts into words and my words into action so that others can learn and share one of the most beautiful and exhilarating experiences they can have and share as I am with you now in a physical lifetime. This is the best way I can express the quintessential definition of unconditional love.

In human terms, we relate this experience in the physical sense as a shock followed by a denial of the experience. Eternal life continues in the connection that never ends. Therefore, to explain this experience holistically will become somewhat easier in the long run. Further, unconditional love would not take human frailty or deterioration of mind and body into account. It just exists. This is what I needed to realize.

As I stated earlier, I do not expect this encounter that I am about to describe in the last two years of Dad's life to be a "religious experience." Although I do respect and love my Roman Catholic religious upbringing, I believe religion to be only a component of spiritual life and a guiding instrument toward totally holistic spiritualism. I view religion as consequential, based on a review of earthly practices by our eternal Creator to determine whether or not we are worthy of entering blissful eternal life. I do not view spiritualism as one God separating one soul from one body at the time of physical death. Rather, at the time of physical death, one God continues as one with the soul through eternity, experiencing what is defined as "unconditional love."

As Dad was continuing to deteriorate mentally and physically, in the last two years of his life, my communication with his physical body was becoming extremely difficult and challenged my faith to great extremes. I could not understand how God could make this wonderful human being compromise his dignity to such a great extreme. It was not right, watching him die like this, deteriorating a little more each day. How could God be a loving God and let this happen? How could He say he loves and cares for us? My anger was so great that I began to resent my faith as look at what I believed about God's love as one big lie. In essence, I was challenging my religious beliefs, which are largely based on tradition taught by our ancestors and handed down over the past several thousand years. Again, this is not a testimonial or a criticism of religion as it stands.

Rather, my statements past and going forward in this book are intended to describe experiences of myself in the last two years of Dad's physical life.

My Roman Catholic religion teaches me that there are three persons in one God. Although I cannot materialistically understand this concept, I accept this as truth . I cannot question what I do not understand. My nature has always been to question what I don't understand. However, my upbringing was not to question what I don't understand in my religion. Rather, accept what I don't understand in my religion as truth and consider it a mystery which will be revealed to me after I die. Alternately, however, I can experience what I cannot explain. Experiences do not need a validation; they just are. I believe this to be the essence of the soul; it just is. The human element is the instrument that allows the soul to connect with another soul as one soul. Each time I visited Dad as his body continued to deteriorate with his mind, his physical communication with me also deteriorated. In the last two years of his life, it was difficult for him to move the muscles in his mouth. He barely had the energy or the ability to communicate with me on a level that I could understand. Often, his words were gibberish and made little or no sense. I became discouraged as my visits became less and less productive in the physical sense, and there was little purpose in trying to communicate with him in a manner that elevated any emotion that stimulated the senses, which is common in normal day-to-day communication.

My Roman Catholic upbringing instilled values in me that were very strong. These values were built on the premise that there are three persons in one God. There is virtually no explanation in the physical sense and how that is possible. It is almost impossible to conceptualize, let alone understand. Yet I believe this to be true because my religion teaches me that it is true. The point here is that I believe something that I cannot explain or even understand, yet I accept this as a large part of my religious foundation. I was also taught that I have a free will and mind of my own and that God gave these things to me.

It is considered a mystery of faith, and I can just accept it, or I can debate it and come to my own conclusions. Either way, I cannot prove it one way or another. I need to make a choice on whether or not to believe it. I look at my dad in his deteriorating physical state, and I choose to believe that he will die soon based on my observation. I also choose to believe whether or not I will lose him forever or he will continue on his journey to eternal life, and I will spiritually connect with him throughout the process. I chose the latter not because I could prove it factually but because I felt and experienced it. As a business management professor, I was trained to always look for validation for my theories and prove my hypothesis. Here I need no validation to experiencing unconditional love for my Dad.

Until Dad became ill, I did not truly understand my spiritual relationship with him. Beyond the physical connection of what we refer to as "humanity," the whole experience still remains an enigma to me.

It has always been stated that the eyes are the windows of the soul. As Dad's condition continued to deteriorate, his speech became more labored and difficult to understand. It was almost as if he were speaking in gibberish. At first I could not accept the fact that I could not understand him. Then I began to just look at him with kindness and understanding by following the example of his caregivers. His caregivers saw conditions of this type every day. Therefore, Dad was no exception. They were trained to cope and deal with Alzheimer's patients. Then I watched the caregivers who stroked his face, held his hand, and wiped the saliva permeating from his lips as he could no longer control his facial muscles or saliva glands. Still, despite the training, it took some pretty special individuals to do this job of caregiving. Yet on some days, despite their efforts, they could not get Dad to respond. They asked me to try when I arrived to visit. I used the same words as I always did to get him to respond: "Dad, it's me, Johnny… I love you!" He would suddenly open his eyes even for thirty seconds and smile at me. Whether or not he recognized me or even understood my voice as his son's, he was familiar enough to respond back to me. This was all I needed.

Once upon a time, there was a young father and a small child that shared an experience that many poets would call a trip into eternity. This is where the translation can get very sticky. It gets sticky because it is very difficult to understand yet so easy to experience. In human life, we are always looking for validation when explaining our feelings to others. We often use phrases such as "Do you know what I mean?" The party receiving the communication, when this question is asked, usually returns a blank stare to the inquiring party. The stare quite frankly indicates there was very little or no understanding in the communication. The transmitter of the message in this instance, no matter how hard he or she tries to explain their experience to the receiver, cannot achieve any validation other than what they are feeling or experiencing at the time they are sending the message. The message is gibberish to the receiver because the feelings off the transmitter cannot be expressed in words. Subsequently, both parties are frustrated, and the conversation usually comes to an end.

The brief example of the father and the young child sharing an experience that simulates a trip to eternity uses the mind, which generates imagination and provides a gateway to the soul that manifests its existence though our feelings or emotions. For example, the experience I had with my father as a small child and the correlation of that experience I described as a "trip to eternity" is raised to a higher level of consciousness that needs no validation except that it exists. This example and experience with my dad as a small child will set the stage for what is to be explained and not validated throughout the remainder of this chapter. You will read and translate into your mind to your own level of understanding how living with Alzheimer's can open your spirit through your mind and use it as an instrument that will provide a gateway to your eternal soul. If your experience is similar to mine, then you will listen and understand with your heart, and it will never cease to beat beyond the boundless confines of your eternal soul. Finally, your trip with Alzheimer's with you or with a loved one will have meaning from this point forward to the end of human life. Although human life will end, eternal life will continue through the eternal soul.

This chapter is not about religion. It is not even about faith associated with "believing." This is not about believing. Rather, it is about what is, has always been, and always will be. I would like to bring the reader back to the mystery of three persons existing in one God. The reader should understand that the narrative to follow is not to provide any validation that there are three persons in one God. Subsequently, there will be no validation provided as to why or how my communication with my dad through the silence of living with the Alzheimer's condition raised me to a higher level of consciousness. This unconditional love that I speak of provided feelings that correlated to the feelings I experienced as a little boy with the younger dad on the Boston Common. Our minds were matched as one mind and one spirit without words or provocation through human silence each time I visited him in the last two years of his human life.

Remembering with the Human Connection

The human element lives in an existence that is governed by time. Time makes everything finite and draws limits to every moment of our existence. You see, everything we do and say has a beginning and an end. The human connection I had with my dad was not concerned with time. Therefore, my memories of him exist in my mind as reminiscence of unconditional love. As discussed earlier in this book, unconditional love is not concerned with time, as it is concerned with the connection of mind, body, and soul. Although this section will not focus on the soul, the incidents that will be mentioned here would not be possible without the soul.

This section will use time as a reference to incidents that occurred that brought special meaning to both Dad and me. I believe life to be a series of incidents that occur between individuals who are brought together by family connections, all who have come together by some other means. The quintessential question is, are these connections made by coincidence or by chance? Does everything happen for a reason? Or do situations occur without provocation or meaning?

When I was eighteen years old, my life involved having good times with my friends, working a part-time job, and going to school. My brother, Ralph, who is seven years my junior, had a very different lifestyle because of our age differences. I remember as a family we would always have our meals together as much as possible, especially on the weekends. Dad would always sit at the head of the table, and we would always say grace before our meals. There were only four of us in our family: Dad, Mother, my brother, and myself. We had a very special bond together, as Dad would always be very quiet while we were eating a meal. His presence and demeanor just had an inexplicable magic about making us believe he had everything under control and that he would always be there for us. He had his favorite dishes that he would ask Mother to make, and she would make them for him. He never complained if the meal was not cooked exactly right or if something was left out of the meal.

I also remember that during our meals we had many discussions of what was happening in our lives at the time. Dad always listened carefully and passionately about what was going on in our lives as if it were going on in his life. Yes, he was a part of our lives, and we knew that. This is what made our family bond so special. As I was growing up, Dad never judged anyone or anything. He would never force his values or beliefs on us to pass judgment or criticize our decisions. He allowed us to make choices based on our experiences rather than his. Dad was not judgmental and allowed my brother and I to make choices yet take responsibility for the consequences. Mother was always included in the discussions at mealtime. She held very strong opinions about what we did. And that is another story in itself. Both my brother and I love our mother. She was a very important part of our upbringing and always will remain in our hearts.

Dad never owned a house. He worked hard every single day of his life. And he very rarely complained about anything, taking all things in stride. When Dad was not around, Mother would often talk about the days when she and Dad first got married. They would live in a very modest apartment just to make ends meet. When going to work each day and a new baby in the household, Dad would have nothing in his pocket except twenty-eight cents for a package of cigarettes and two cents to buy a newspaper. He would bring a boxed lunch to work in an industrial-sized lunchbox and would be perfectly happy. Again, he never complained. Yes, Dad was a simple man who led his household in a very loving manner. I am not speaking about the simplicity of how he lived his life as one would normally interpret the word *simple*. I interpret *simple* as meaning "transparent." Dad became one with our lives, as opposed to his life being a separate entity when compared to our lives as a family. Here he was with two young children and the young wife who lived very different lifestyles while he was working each day. When we sat down for supper each evening, we would usually begin with a small prayer. I remember that after saying grace, we would all discuss what happened in our lives that day. Dad would sit quietly and listen and never passed judgment on what we said or did that day. He would always talk about his day last. He would blend his day into our day as if we were all together, yet doing different things.

I remember one evening coming home from elementary school. I think I was in the eighth grade. I got three Cs and an F on my report card and needed it signed by both my parents. I was petrified to show my dad and had already been scolded and grounded by my mom. She said what is typically said by a mom with a child who got a bad report card. She said, "Wait until your father gets home!" My father did get home, and we all ate supper in the same manner as we always did and started with a prayer of thanksgiving.

Then we all talked about our day and, as I stated earlier, Dad always went last. When it was my turn, I actually told him about my report card, figuring it would come up sooner or later. Dad just looked at me and didn't say anything and continued to eat. Then he asked my brother about his day. I really thought he was going to lash out when he heard about my report card, and he didn't. Before I went to bed that night, he came into my bedroom, and I was doing my homework. He tucked me in as he always did and had returned the report card back to me, signed. He smiled at me and said, "I already talked to your mother about this, and just do better." That was how he responded to the bad report card. He addressed things simply and to the point and never elaborated on what was already addressed. This is what I admired about him. He set the tone for love though trust in our family, and it worked. One could say that Dad's spirituality kept us together rather than separated us, although we were all doing different things in the course of the day.

This author would also venture to say that the most prominent psychological analysts would have to write novels explaining the effectiveness and validity of Dad's lifestyle as a very "simple" man. Perhaps it can be stated as a lesson to learn from what was just described above that gentleness and compassion, more importantly understanding, raises this author to a different level of consciousness in living his lifestyle that was taught by Dad so many years ago. Dad simplicity was nurtured form the love he had for his family that never ended when he got Alzheimer's. His love, it just continued even if he could not physically communicate that to us. The rationale was that love was not a condition of give and take. Rather, Dad treated love as simple and transparent as a lifestyle he shared with us as one family. The point here is that we were one and not four separate parts in our family.

Dad spoke little at the kitchen table but became one with our thoughts and our minds. Just by his presence, his demeanor rendered a certain comfort level that allowed us to express ourselves anyway we chose using both body language and expressive conversation. This type of behavior was uncommon in the middle to late '60s and early '70s when we grew up. The best way to express how Dad integrated with our family was to describe how his life differentiated with ours in the course of the day and later incorporated with us when we were together in the evening at dinner time. We were separate, yet we were one as a family.

Jumping ahead, I also recall an incident in my life that showed Dad's great love for every member of my family. Dad did not play favorites, and treated me and my brother the same. He loved us both the same and was never biased on his decisions regarding our welfare and his judgment on the decisions that we made. In fact, he rarely freely stated in words, "I love you." Dad would just look at us and say, "I love you," with his eyes. All Dad had to do was look at us, and we knew that we had love. When I announced to my family that I was getting married, Dad responded with no words, but his eyes showed great joy. He looked at me and my future wife, Gale, with such intensity and love that it made me want to cry. It was his look that rendered great understanding, and there was no condition to the love it represented. This represented his successes as a parent and the choice made by my future wife and me to become one in holy matrimony. He then consummated our announcement with a toast to our future success as husband and wife.

The key point to the preceding paragraph is that Dad consummated our marriage intentions and was not a priest. He acknowledged Gale and me as one, and he became part of that union between her and me. The human connection as we know it had a certain consciousness related to it that could not be expressed in words, only in thought and mind. The recognition of the union between two bodies as one entity serves as the conduit of communication that relates to an eternal existence.

The final example I would like to discuss in this section describing the human connection is one that is very special and dear to my heart. In June of 1997, I was having fun with my son at my parents' home in East Boston. My son was only seven years of age at the time, and I was throwing him on the counter in the kitchen and then placing him gently on the kitchen floor. After repeating this motion several times, I felt a strange sensation in my chest, one that I had never felt before. I thought that perhaps the sensation was caused by some misalignment of my muscle structure and quickly discounted the pain as minor in nature. Although the repetitive motion had ceased, the sensation in my chest never really left me. In fact, it got worse every time I walked and then stopped walking. Remaining in denial that there was anything seriously wrong with me, I decided to go to the doctor and ask him to do some manipulation on my skeletal structure to avoid getting this pain in my chest.

Wisely, the doctor decided to give me an EKG. Rather than manipulation, the doctor decided to examine my heart first. He obviously did not like what he heard and what he read on the EKG tape. He decided to send me to the hospital for a stress test as soon as possible. The stress test was positive, and I was immediately scheduled for surgery. That week, I found myself on a stretcher and ready to receive two stents inserted into my heart to keep my arteries open. The evening before surgery, I lived the longest day of my life. Every moment that went by, I lived that dread of not having to be lucky enough to survive the surgery. I remembered that evening talking to every family member for hours. I could not fall asleep despite the heavy sedation I was under. I wanted to run out of the hospital and escape this entire horrible nightmare that I was reliving over and over again. I remember talking to my dad, and he simply said to me, "Do not worry, son. Everything will be okay."

Dad's voice was very gentle, yet very firm and convincing. He stated that I would be okay with assertiveness as well as compassion. His voice was kind but convincing, assertive yet demanding results of success. Yes, this was the same, simple dad that I had known all my life that spoke to me with his body through the eternal the soul. The end result was I was okay. A few weeks later after my surgery, mother shared with me that after Dad hung up my call to him before my surgery, he said the same thing as his dad said when he was eighteen years old, lying in a foxhole on Normandy Beach in France during World War II. His dad said, as my dad also said, "If you are going to take him, take me instead and spare him." Dad was spared. I was also spared. However, Dad was not taken back in 1997 when I had my surgery. The end result was that my grandfather died of a cerebral hemorrhage when Dad was eighteen years old, fighting for his country while lying in a foxhole during World War II. Dad died thirteen years after my surgery. In fact, Dad answered the call to join the Armed Forces on May 3, 1943, and passed away May 3, 2010. When delivering his eulogy on May 6, 2010, I made it a point to bring out the fact that Dad joined the armed forces over sixty-seven years ago, protecting his country. I found myself delivering his eulogy after five and a half years of watching him being cared for by the armed forces personnel in the veterans' hospital.

In closing this chapter, President John F. Kennedy's Inaugural Speech, January 20, 1961, comes to mind. He said, "Ask not what your country can do for you. Rather, ask what you can do for your country."

There is no doubt in my mind that this country took care of Dad in the last years of his human life, and rightfully so, as Dad took care of his country when it needed him. This is what I remember in my human connection with Dad.

Validating with the Spiritual Connection

This integration holds all the secrets of the universe, seen and unseen, discovered and not known on a conscious level. However, all of these elements described above, known and not known, exist in the eternal essence of the divine Creator. What has just been stated is the belief through the perceptions of the author who has spent the majority of his life researching, in linear sequential terms, how theories translate into facts that are measurable and observable in finite terms. In other words, I may not be able to logically explain many of my feelings.

I believe that feelings need no validation. Rather, they are the windows to the soul and relate to some common bond or more experience in eternal communication through the unification of mind, body, and spirit. The silence that I speak of here specifically relates to that communication with my dad. Therefore, it is through listening in silence to all of these sounds communicated through pure energy within the brilliant existence of our eternal Creator will serve as the only needed validation to this narration. Only the silence will count, and life eternal will become the only reality that has been felt by this author. What is to follow will be a last communication of the human element with Dad over the past two years of Dad's human earthly existence and the continuance of the eternal communication one with the eternal Creator.

Since early June of 2008, it became quite apparent that Dad's physical condition was rapidly deteriorating. He could barely make cohesive sentences from this point forward. He could not walk on his own, having been wheelchair-bound for the past three years. Every time he looked at me, it would take him incredible efforts to make a sentence with his mouth and focus his eyes on my face. His facial muscles would curl and tighten when trying to form words, even when attempting something simple such as crack a smile. However, there was something special in his being, which made him desire a communication with me at some higher level of consciousness. At this time, I did not realize or understand what he was trying to do. My frustration was increasing at this time with each passing visit. Nothing would change, and sometimes when I would visit him, he would be in his wheelchair, awake but not able to open his eyes. He would be mumbling some type of gibberish that I did not understand. He would then move his hands forward and backward in a circular motion while his facial muscles were tensing and relaxing, trying to communicate with me.

I would feel this incredible burst of emotion within my being and a desire to lash out in anger and frustration to what I was experiencing at this time with my father. After several attempts at trying to justify the validity of my experiences with each successful painful visit, I became disillusioned because my inner being was being destroyed. My personal religious values began to clash with my experiences with Dad and watching him die physically. I could not understand how any god or supreme being allowed this to happen to such a wonderful man who dedicated his life to his family and his friends and, most importantly, to his God. I could not understand how a man who fought for his country and asked for nothing in return could suffer in such a manner. It appears that all of his dignity had been robbed of him. This man was not able to move his bowels on his own, bound to a wheelchair, and had little or no visitors each day. I believed at that time that this was a tragedy of the human being that I once knew. I needed a validation of this experience, and I needed it here and now. I never got that validation and became increasingly frustrated and angry.

I would go into work every day with a shattered spirit and a smile on my face. What I was feeling was a contradiction to what I was showing to the world. The smile on my face was masking the inner conflict of anger and frustration simply because it was necessary. My waking hours became a living hell because I was trying to be something I was not. My spirit was not in sync with my body. Often my workers and colleagues would ask me if I was okay when they saw me alone in my office with my head in my hands. I told them I was fine and just taking a little break. They just smiled at me and kept walking. Apparently I needed this validation of what I was experiencing. I was not finding one. There was apparently no validation to this human experience that was shaking my spirit in such a manner that it made me forget who I was more than remember what I was doing. I was trying to validate my own existence and why my role as Dad's primary caretaker as a family member was justified. I was seeking an answer from some god who was putting me through this awful torment and making me realize my own mortality was worth very little. I viewed these visits with Dad as punitive and consequential to some sins I may have committed in my lifetime. Yes, I felt this was my punishment or retribution to my own life. It apparently was all about me and not about Dad. I did not realize this at the time until just before his death.

Perhaps as time went on between 2008 and 2010, I began to realize my own mortality and depended on Dad to provide the answers to why I was feeling the way I did. I asked this question over and over until late 2008. In November of 2008, I noticed that Dad was responding to me less and less each day, physically that is. Observing this deterioration was almost unbearable. I began creating many excuses as to why they did not want to go to see him. I even came up with the justification in my mind of not seeing him that I would compare my behavior to that of my family and friends and state to myself, "I cannot really bear to see him this way." At the time, I did not see this as a copout, but rather as a justification of my own mortality.

I remember around Thanksgiving in 2008 that I was gathering my thoughts about why I should not go and see Dad for the holidays. I remember around that time how I would make excuses about people that I came in contact with that had colds or the flu and that I had contracted their germs. This would give me a justification of how I may have been carrying the germ or had contracted the germ myself and how I could have made Dad very ill by visiting him. I also justified that he could not verbalize his discomfort when contracting these germs and how they could kill them if the nurses did not know he was ill. I was totally disillusioned and not really confident that this was the case. My inner being was lying to myself. However, I could never escape my feelings of alienation from him and intense guilt from not seeing him.

One morning, I remember calling my mother and telling her on my way to work that I was not going to see Dad because my students in my class I was teaching were ill and that I might carry the germ into Dad if I saw him. My mother perfectly understood and advised me not to see him. I felt comforted by her words but tremendously guilty at the same time. On my way to work, I was driving a path that would take me right by the veterans' hospital, where Dad was staying. As I drove closer and closer to the VA, I felt increasingly guilty for not stopping in to see him. I felt so guilty that tears came to my eyes. Rather than drive by the VA, I just drove into the parking lot near the building where Dad was staying, and I sat in my car for about ten minutes. I then justified in my mind that I should drive away and go directly to work. I proceeded to start the car and began to drive away from the VA when something stopped me in my tracks. I suddenly felt this surge of energy and comfort. I now had the strength to go into the VA and visit Dad, taking whatever consequences and responsibility for my actions.

As I drove back into the parking lot, I rationalized in my mind that I should see Dad. However, I should observe him from a distance and not go into his room. I felt that if I spoke loud enough, he could still hear my voice. This made me feel very confident but at the same time lessened my guilt for not seeing him. When I walked through the entrance to the part of the building where Dad was staying, my pace was abrupt as it always is when I walk in to see him. I then turned the corner and walked through the double doors leading to his room. The door to his room was closed, and I had to get to work. I heard much activity going on inside his room and knocked on the door. I observed two nurse assistants who were changing him and getting him ready to go for breakfast. I noticed that his face was a little red. His eyes were closed, and he was making rapid circular motions with his hands. He was trying to communicate with the nurse assistants but had much difficulty communicating. I could see that he was in much distress mentally. He appeared to be fine physically. However, I picked up a signal from him in the form of a feeling, nothing of which I have ever felt before in any of my visits with Dad. The feeling was deep, yet it was transparent and in sync with my feelings. The connection between Dad and me was deep, and I could feel his being, his essence, his soul. Although observing from a distance, I could sense his restlessness and his inability to be free of this physical, tormented condition. His spiritual being seemed to conflict with his physical self, and they were not in sync with one another.

The strange part of this whole observation and what I was experiencing during this visit was so unique and special that I did not question it. Nor was I afraid of it. I just felt this essence of complete connection with my dad. The feeling made me one with him, and I could now begin to understand why he existed, and it was not just to lay in that bed he was in and be tormented because his physical body was disconnected with his soul. In a matter of a few seconds, I now began to feel yet not have the ability to rationalize or validate the eternal and perfect manifestation of the human soul. Our observation is that we see them both as one and feel deep sorrow and even remorse from what we are observing at the time. This is perfectly natural and normal. Yet what I am explaining at this point is that this observation on this day validated my connection with my father that I had over the past fifty years in a very special way.

When I speak of understanding the spiritual connection using the example cited in the previous paragraph, I do not refer to understanding in the traditional sense but rather understanding as an acceptance of what is rather than what we want it to be. It is not up to humanity to understand why the design of existence by our eternal Creator is unclear. Rather, it is to be accepted as what is, has always been, and will always be. There are no words to express this feeling in its entirety. You just have to experience it. Do not try to understand or validate its existence. Just feel it! You will find that what you feel is complete joy and radiant energy that gives hope to the loved one being observed in a physical state of torment.

In a matter of a few seconds, my whole life changed because I believed and did not rationalize. I understood and did not validate. I felt unconditional love, which I accepted yet did not ask for, because I was one with my soul, mind, and body with my dad. Although our bodies were in different physical states, their connections with our souls eliminated any diseased states of physical being. In other words, spiritual connections are not tied to physical matter. At the time this event occurred back in 2008, I experienced unconditional love for the first time with my dad. This was pure, unadulterated love that could only be experienced and not communicated physically, only spiritually. It was an experience like no other ever felt, seen, or heard. It was just simply amazing. I was so humbled by what I felt I immediately said good-bye to the nurses' assistants and left the building where Dad was staying. I left with such a feeling of contentment and completeness that my mind could not conceive to understand as it interpreted impulses traveling through my senses into fresh thoughts in what I had just experienced. They were just no words to describe what just happened.

Each subsequent visit to my dad became less difficult as he continued to degenerate physically in both mind and body. At one point, our family had a meeting with the doctors at the VA who basically told us that Dad's condition was deteriorating rapidly and we should prepare for the worst over the next several months. It became increasingly difficult since Christmas of 2008 and Christmas of 2010 for my mother to visit my dad in his degenerating state. However, I felt it was my duty and obligation to continue to see Dad as much as I could each day since I was the closest one to him demographically and the oldest son. I believed as long as I could continue to make this connection with Dad's innermost being that the observation of his degenerating mind and body would not affect me as much as before I made that connection. I would be able to persevere as his primary connection in the DiCicco Family.

Communicating
in Silence

The power that I speak of is not forceful or demanding. Rather, it identifies a raised level of consciousness that embodies pure communication with the eternal Creator in union with the immortal soul. The soul of which I refer speaks of a union rather than a separation of consciousness between Dad and me. I can remember back to January of 2009, right around Dad's eighty-fourth birthday, while he was in a degenerating physical state and could hardly form words that I could understand. I built my best communication with him through unconditional love. This was the only way I could continue to visit him in his physical state and consider our meeting together productive.

I had the privilege of seeing Dad almost every day since the beginning of 2009. Each visit produced another reason rather than an excuse to plan another visit. I discovered that I was learning about my own existence as much as my dad's through this communication. I also discovered that we were not different in our spiritual connection, and we were unified spiritually with the eternal Creator through unconditional love.

What is communicating in silence? What is seen and not heard? What is love without physical expression? What is a faith that is not consequential? Finally, what is believed and not seen? There is no sequence to these questions, nor is there any logic that validates them. We cannot create any hypotheses or draw assumptions that will validate answers to any of these questions. Therefore, what is the point about writing on anything that cannot provide validation or logic? One would say it is a leap of faith. Others would say there is no point. I simply state that writing about his experience is simply what experienced together and because of that experience, it became unconditional without need for validation other than it took place. I was a part of Dad. and it has been and will always be that way. Therefore, if I loved him unconditionally, then he loved me unconditionally.

One morning in January of 2009 right after Dad's eighty-fourth birthday, I had a rather unusual visit with Dad. He just finished getting cleaned up and was all dressed and ready to go for breakfast. The nursing assistants knew I was there to see him and did not have much time, so they left his room. I was now alone with Dad and making friendly conversation with him in a cheerful manner as I always did each morning I visited him. During this time, I was fiddling around with his TV set to try to get the volume higher. I was not looking at his face and only concentrating on the TV.

My back was turned away from him, and I heard some sounds coming from his wheelchair that did not make any sense at all. I then turned to look at Dad, and his face appeared to be quite red, and his eyes were tightly closed as he was making rapid circular motions with his hands. His fists were clenched tightly, and he was continuing to make gibberish sounds that made absolutely no sense at all.

There was something different about the sounds that he was making from the time my back was turned away from him and then began fiddling with the TV set. Although these sounds were the same in frequency, tone, and intensity from when I was fiddling with the TV, they were giving me different messages now as I turned back to look at Dad directly. How could this be? It made absolutely no sense. Yet, I knew there was a difference. Better still, to state it more accurately, I felt there was a difference. There was a difference here that I could not explain. I felt like I was going mad because I did not understand how to interpret my feelings. I felt like I was one with him and I could understand his soul, his very being.

The experience I was having provided a level of communication that was telepathic in nature yet growing with intensity through each passing second I was spending with Dad that morning. The feeling was almost an extension of pre-existing feelings I had for my father that have always been with me, maybe even before I was born. I know this sounds crazy, but I felt his being in union with mine. The communication was different in that the sounds that I heard were gibberish only because I could not and refused to understand him physically on that level. Yet, I could understand him telepathically on a higher conscious level. The conduit between the gibberish communication and the higher level of telepathic consciousness I believe was unconditional love. Ironically, there was no validation I needed for the gibberish words I was hearing. The only validation I needed was the telepathic consciousness I was feeling. As I looked at Dad, directly at his body, making the circular motions with his hands and uttering gibberish words I could not understand, I felt his being in union with mine in such a way that I could see beyond the physical connection with him and me through unconditional love. This unconditional love became a validation of being rather than understanding. I now knew him for what he is, rather than remembered him for what he was physically—one time ago.

The telepathy I was feeling sent a message that provided clear communication of agreement, not in words, but in essence of being. It was a covenant that validates the spirit as one with God, which comprises the very essence of existence. You see, Dad was telling me to understand that his spirit could not be tarnished or affected by physical pain or mental anxiety. The telepathy sent a clear message that his physical body was not giving me the same message as his spiritual being. This is not to state that this represented disconnect between body and soul. Rather, it validates the unity between both and the different messages they were sending concurrently. Once realizing this, I felt this incredible warmth going through my whole body that enlightened my mind to what I was experiencing in just a few seconds that seemed like an eternity. I could now see and feel beyond the gibberish and into my father's consciousness for the first time since I have known him. Yes, I was him, and he was me, and we were connected with God for all time. I consider this feeling to be a gift of his spiritual consciousness rather than a gift of faith. I was not forced to believe what I was feeling. I just know I felt this. I did not have to seek it because it was already there. I did not have to ask for it in prayer because it was already there. Yes, I realized what I had just experienced needed no logic or explanation to validate any more than the existence of God.

——•——

On Easter Sunday 2009, I remembered driving my mother to see my dad at the Brockton VA. I remember picking up my wife and taking her with me to Sunday mass at the VA with Mom. When we got to see Dad, he was absolutely radiant. Dad was smiling from one ear to the other. He truly appeared happy to see us all. My son was also with us that day. Dad was not usually in such high spirits. This was a special day for all of us. He could not stop smiling at us. Dad was so excited he was moving his feet up and down in very rapid motions yet found it difficult to lift his leg. I remember him trying to say words. However, they came out very gibberish really and not easy to understand at all. His hands continued to reach out to each of us as he tried to touch us. We got closer so he could run his hands up and down our clothing and he could feel us. This was a very special day indeed. [Note to layout: insert photo 01]

I remember taking Dad to mass, holding onto his wheelchair and fixing my eyes on the wheels of his vehicle as they were going around. I felt something really strange, although Dad was not saying anything. I turned to look at him, and his eyes were now clamped shut. His hands were still moving in a circular motion, yet he was not saying anything. I was puzzled yet somewhat intrigued in what I was observing. However, the strange feeling I had inside would not go away. In fact, it intensified. When we arrived at mass, one floor up from Dad's room at the VA, Dad was fast asleep. His hands were no longer moving in a circular motion. His feet were not going up and down, and his eyes were still clenched tight. However, the strange feeling I had did not go away. In fact, it was continuing to intensify. For some strange reason, I felt that Dad was still aware of what was going on around him. I felt it, but his body sent a different message. He was not responding to my verbal requests to wake up. How could that be? My emotions made no sense at all. There was so much noise at the time it was amazing how Dad was sleeping through all of this. More amazing was that in the strangest way, I still felt like I was communicating with him. I was really confused but didn't say anything to anyone.

Dad had slept through the homily of the mass and even began to snore during the offertory part of the mass. Then suddenly, during the recital of the Our Father prayer, Dad began to recite the prayer with us. Although the prayer he was reciting was gibberish, I could understand the words he was trying to say. His

John DiCicco

eyes were still clamped shut. However, his lips were moving in a very rapid motion until the prayer ended. The Our Father was his favorite prayer. Somehow he remembered this prayer, and the familiarity with the words allowed him to come out of a deep sleep and pray with us. This is not what was intriguing about this whole experience. The intensified feeling of communicating with Dad, although his eyes were clamped down tightly shut, now ended when Dad began to recite the Our Father prayer. I can't explain why. My silent telepathic communication with him was interrupted while in the silence of his physical being when he physically began to recite the prayer.

I then realized that I was communicating with Dad on a totally different level than I have ever communicated with him before at such a higher and better level of consciousness. My consciousness with him was spiritual, much more than it was physical before he began to recite the prayer. In other words, Dad and I were reciting the Our Father prayer together as one, telepathically, before we physically recited the prayer at mass as a group with my family and the rest of the congregation who were present that day. I wanted to share this experience with the reader, not because I was trying to make sense of it, but rather to relate how unconditional love unites the soul without experiencing physical or emotional pain. It is in every sense of the word *creation*. Yes, Dad and I created consciousness through prayer that defies and even negates physical or emotional pain that is representative of human mortality. For a fleeting moment while at mass, we could actually experience our own existence as one with the eternal Creator. After reciting the Our Father prayer, Dad fell back to sleep, and the intense emotion I felt earlier disappeared.

Living through the Eyes of the Soul

Growing up as a child, I was also taught that God was a circle, as he had no beginning and no end, and additionally, I was also taught that my soul was immortal and will live forever. I really don't know what the soul looks like. In fact, I don't even know what an angel looks like. I do know that we try to give spiritual beings human qualities so that we can understand them better through the use of our senses. It appears that what we don't understand, we assign human traits to identify physical characteristics to spiritual beings to make valued judgments such as good or evil. This clearly is not what this book is about, as it contains no consequences, makes no assumptions of good or evil, or, most importantly, does not try to judge the soul based on a person's life, particularly my dad's life.

I can no more explain eternity any more than I can explain how an entire nervous system comprised of millions of complex parts fits into an ant. What I do know is that what I do not understand often does make a lot of sense. I believe that the soul is what makes us human. I also believe that what makes us who we are and defines our characteristics as human beings is much more than DNA. Our souls define us as who we are rather than what we were or what we will become. There might be a very good reason why an Alzheimer's patient is stuck in the same time period. These individuals are living their purpose as opposed to defining their purpose for living. They say that Alzheimer's is the deterioration of the brain, and the patient slowly loses touch with reality and eventually loses his or her capacity to perform basic bodily functions. Loved ones experience a horrendous transformation of an individual they once knew and loved, remotely evaluating them from a physical or emotional standpoint.

From a loved one's viewpoint, the emotional pain of coping with this rapid deterioration of mind and body in which there is no known cure becomes extremely difficult to handle. I watched my dad deteriorate almost five and a half years physically and mentally. Many days I found it almost impossible to understand how a loving God can allow this type of thing to happen to someone I care for so much. Dad did not have a mean bone in his body. He always reached out to help others. He always put himself last and others first so that they could be the winners and he could be the conduit that provided for them. My human characteristics emotionally drained my spirit and my soul to the point where I was angered at my Creator because He allowed such a good man that he should suffer as much as he did in the last five and a half years of his life.

As I continue to ponder how Dad was such a victim of such a cruel disease, which would eventually result in the termination of his life, I began to think about Jesus. I didn't think of Jesus as the "Son of God." I thought of him as a historic figure that others believed was the Son of God who gave his life for his friends. Jesus never wrote a book, had a building erected in his name, or declared himself any different than those who surrounded him. He called his friends "brothers." He allowed himself to be crucified and while in the process (as history records) asked his Creator to forgive those who crucified him because they did not know what they were doing. Jesus had reached that higher level of consciousness where he could forgive those who trespassed against him beyond his physical and emotional pain of the cruelest nature on the day of his crucifixion. He gave his life for his friends.

Based on the aforementioned, suffering may be, whether physical or emotional or both, a relative experience perceived through our senses within a certain time restraint. In retrospect, the soul doesn't experience the physical components of suffering. In the Creator's infinite wisdom, he decided that the human element could integrate with the soul, which is at a higher level of consciousness. We call this higher level of consciousness "feelings."

Just as the body is stimulated through the senses, the soul is stimulated through the consciousness of being. From a pragmatic standpoint in applying humanistic terms to the soul, feelings—our communication with the soul—are evident in what we refer to as *emotions*. Emotions have no base of validity and no justification for existence. They are evident without explanation and manifest themselves through the eyes of the soul. The human element cannot deny that emotions exist. Science, however, has identified various parts of the brain where emotions are generated. However, there is no explanation as to how they formulate a rationalization to explain labeled feelings such as "love," "hate," "joy," or "sorrow." These are the elements generated from the soul. This is what makes us who we are and what we have always been at a higher level of consciousness.

John DiCicco

Unconditional Love
of the Soul

I find the word *love* to be a very powerful word containing multifaceted meanings. Many times we find ourselves telling people that are close to us that we love them. We use the word *love* spontaneously, sometimes without even realizing its meaning. However, using the word *love* signifies an emotion of unparalleled caring.

There has been so much written about the word *love* over the centuries. However, it has always been and will always be an emotion relating to a mutual feeling of completeness and acceptance. There are literally hundreds of thousands of literary pieces written about the word *love*. Words such as *kind*, *unselfish*, *caring*, and *everlasting* represents only a few of the synonyms that describe the word. However, the point is that love is something that is not tangible. We can't touch it, we can't smell it, and we can't see it. However, we can feel it. In fact, some of us will even die for love.

In light of the previous two paragraphs, what is this emotion we call love, really? Where does it come from? Why does it exist in us? Why does something so powerful need no validation or explanation to justify its existence? Most importantly, why will some of us even sacrifice our lives for it? History tells us that Jesus sacrificed his life for his friends on the cross at Calvary over two thousand years ago. It is recorded he did this because he loves us. We have been following his teachings for over two thousand years, which resounds the meanings of true love.

It is recorded in history that Jesus had and an "unconditional love" for all humanity. It is also recorded that as Jesus was hanging from the cross just before he expired, he looked up to his heavenly Father and asked that he forgive the people that crucified him because they knew not what they were doing. If this recording is factually true, then this is a clear indication that Jesus was communicating at a higher conscious level. He was communicating on a level that we could not understand unless we were at the same place that Jesus was at the time of his crucifixion. Whether you believe Jesus to be the Son of God, a great prophet, or someone who has evolved to a higher level of consciousness and has come back to express the meaning of true spirituality of the soul, we can learn so much from his teachings and example. It is also recorded that when Jesus took his last breath, he looked up to his heavenly Father and asserted that his mission had been fulfilled and is finished.

Putting all the pieces of the puzzle together here, it would appear that the spirit was separate from the physical pain Jesus was feeling at the time of his crucifixion. This spirit was communicated to the Father, and the Father was communicating his essence to the Son. However, the mystery of faith translates that the Father and the Son were one with the Spirit. Hence the mystery of the trinity, which I have mentioned several times in this narrative, now has a true purpose toward redemption. Jesus was able and willing to endure his crucifixion because, although his physical life was ending, his spiritual life was continuing, and his soul was glorified through the Holy Spirit. The communion with the Holy Spirit was the essence that provided the conduit of transparency that existed between the Father and the Son. This was the greatest example of unconditional love through the unity of the Spirit that joins all of us in existence eternal.

Getting back to Dad in the last stages of his Alzheimer's condition at the Brockton Veterans Hospital, it was apparent that Dad's physical pain and suffering was separate from his spiritual presence. When I went to visit him, what I saw wasn't necessarily what was going on with his soul. It is my belief that Dad's soul wanted to leave a body, which no longer communicated with family and friends. I cannot rationalize this is what Dad felt. All I know is when I looked at him, he spoke to me through his eyes. His eyes told me that he was ready to go to the next level. His eyes told me that he was tired; his eyes told me that there was something much better, which was waiting for him. No, he didn't physically verbalize this to me. He didn't have the ability to move his facial muscles so that they could form words any longer. Yet I understood.

Just as I cannot explain the love I felt for my father, I could not explain how I was able to communicate with him through the silence, telling me that he was ready to be raised to a higher level of consciousness. However, the only way I would be able to understand what he was saying to me in the silence, I too would also have to rise to that higher level of consciousness so that my spirit could meet his in the process. This experience can only be achieved through the spirituality that exists with unconditional love. This is love that cannot be compromised or forfeited at any time. Is eternal love that has no beginning and has no end; it just is.

Unconditional Love of the Eternal Soul through the Alzheimer's Experience

This book really isn't about Dad, and it isn't about me, the author. It is about all of us who are going through this horrific physical experience we refer to as "Alzheimer's disease." The emotional pain I experienced when I looked at Dad's wretched body deteriorating in mind and physical appearance is like a gray, wintry day. However, until I realized what was really going on, I was not at peace with myself or anybody else around me. About three weeks before Dad passed away, I experienced a huge awakening of why I existed and he existed in the Creator's eternal plan. After I had my annual physical in April 2010, I realized my soul was one with Dad and only could be realized through unconditional love. I truly believe that you cannot experience good until you experience evil. I truly believe that you cannot experience life until you witness death.

I truly believe you cannot understand unconditional love until you experience it. I never realized how much I knew about my father until I experienced the unconditional love that was permeating from his soul.

I could tell my dad how much I loved him. I could feel emotion when I talked to him or about him, which I thought was love. However, I could not experience the unconditional love of his soul until I separated his physical being from his spiritual self. This was shortly after the doctor had asked me if my feelings for my father were selfish ones. This stopped me in my tracks, and I realized that I was so focused on my feelings on my well being and my future without him that I became detached rather than connected to my dad. I also realized that I could never ever connect with my dad again in the way I wanted until I had closure with him. This closure I am writing about was physical before his physical passing. I needed to connect prior to his physical passing to continue my journey with him spiritually. The only instrument that I had to work with was the instrument of love that is unconditional love. This love needed no validation or excuses. It held no pain or sorrow. It did, however, require compassion and understanding. Dad held on to his physical life for over nine days without food or water until our entire family was there at his bedside, wishing farewell from his earthly existence.

I remember the last day of Dad's physical life. I got a phone call from my brother while teaching an evening course on May 3, 2010. Then my brother said that Dad was stable and holding his own, and he was going to jog with his wife, and my mother was going to socialize with some neighbors in her apartment. I felt relieved when getting this call, and I continued to teach for about an hour. That evening when I left school, I was driving home peacefully when, unexpectedly, I received a call from the Brockton Veteran's Hospital. The call came from a Dr. Chin. The doctor stated that Dad had passed away at approximately 7:40 that evening. I immediately took control of the situation and telephoned my son to go to my mom's house where my brother and sister-in-law were staying. I was relieved and saddened at the same time but knew Dad would no longer be in a wretched physical state and his soul would be glorified to a higher level of consciousness. Yes, the soul that I connected with through unconditional love, love experiencing the atrocities of this dreaded disease.

Unconditional Love of the Eternal Creator through the Soul

I believe that everyone is born into this world for a reason. I believe that every creature, every grain of sand, every star in the universe, and all human beings have a purpose. I believe that we are one with the eternal Creator, as he is one with us. I also believe that there is no existence in our known universe that would create life to destroy it or not give it hope. I believe that life is a gift from our eternal Creator in which we coexist for the greater good.

Alzheimer's is a dreaded, despicable, emotionally painful physical disease that robs the mind and the body of physical and mental capacities. However, it does not have the ability to blemish the soul even one little bit. Experiencing Alzheimer's made me realize one very beautiful thing throughout the five-years-plus I watched my father physically and mentally deteriorate: I realize that he will always be with me in spirit, and what I was experiencing through my senses wasn't what was going on at a higher conscious level. I realized a very special closeness with my Creator, as one with my dad and as one with all the Creator's creatures in this universe. I realize that all of us are connected in a very special way, which could not be created or destroyed because they have always existed through our eternal Creator. Most importantly, I realized that the Creator cannot exist without us, and we cannot exist without the Creator, as we are one through eternity.

Afterword

There is very little that can be explained about Alzheimer's that translates into anything that is physically encouraging. It is a devastating disease that robs the mind and the body of a meaningful living existence. It is equally devastating and emotionally draining for the victim's families to watch their loved ones virtually deteriorate to the point where they can no longer sustain day-to-day functioning on their own. The entire process is mentally challenging for all parties concerned, including the caretakers of the victims. Science has experienced some major breakthroughs on what causes this dreaded disease genetically but really has not concretely established how to prevent or cure this disease.

I believe this book in some small way can help support the efforts of those trying to cope with this disease through the realization that what is seen through the senses may be not all that is going on through this journey.

I have never and will never lose the spiritual essence of my dad, as we have and always will be one through the eternal Creator. In essence, to try to justify why God allows pain and suffering to exist in our world would be to separate our Creator from the pain and suffering. He or she is as much of the pain and suffering as we are…all connected as one. Further, it is impossible to put the camel through the eye of a needle, as it is impossible to experience joy and exhilaration without experiencing pain and suffering. The soul is alienated from pain and suffering of the wretched body when it decides to leave that body and go to that higher level of consciousness. This can only be achieved in union with our eternal Creator, who can only exist in us through unconditional love.

Love is much more than just faith. It is much more than just an emotion. Love is the essence of pure energy that is felt through the everlasting power of the soul. The soul lives in the Creator of all things, and the only nourishment that it needs is the acceptance of its existence. Whether you communicate with your loved one on a conscious or telepathic level, their soul gets the message loud and clear. I can attest to this without validation because I have nothing to prove, only to witness.

Finally, understand that there is no such word as *final* or *terminal* when it comes to the soul. You see, unconditional love, as the soul and the Creator are one, just is, always has, and will be…the alpha and the omega through eternity.